Nicky,

You are Love!
This is all.
   Keep Shining.

   Love, Love, Love

   Danielle Miller

[handwritten note, mirror-reversed]

You are loved!
Love, Love, Love,

CONDUIT OF LIGHT

CHANNELED WISDOM FROM OUR HIGHEST CONSCIOUSNESS FOR THE SEEKER OF WELLNESS AND SPIRITUAL FREEDOM

DANIELLE WILKINSON

BALBOA.
PRESS
A DIVISION OF HAY HOUSE

Balboa Press books may be ordered through booksellers or by contacting:

Balboa Press
A Division of Hay House
1663 Liberty Drive
Bloomington, IN 47403
www.balboapress.com
1 (877) 407-4847

Because of the dynamic nature of the Internet, any web addresses or links contained in this book may have changed since publication and may no longer be valid. The views expressed in this work are solely those of the author and do not necessarily reflect the views of the publisher, and the publisher hereby disclaims any responsibility for them.

The author of this book does not dispense medical advice or prescribe the use of any technique as a form of treatment for physical, emotional, or medical problems without the advice of a physician, either directly or indirectly. The intent of the author is only to offer information of a general nature to help you in your quest for emotional and spiritual well-being. In the event you use any of the information in this book for yourself, which is your constitutional right, the author and the publisher assume no responsibility for your actions.

Any people depicted in stock imagery provided by Getty Images are models, and such images are being used for illustrative purposes only. Certain stock imagery © Getty Images.

Print information available on the last page.

ISBN: 978-1-9822-0546-1 (sc)
ISBN: 978-1-9822-0545-4 (e)

Library of Congress Control Number: 2018906809

Balboa Press rev. date: 08/15/2018

DEDICATIONS

This book is dedicated to my loving husband Ken who has been a passenger alongside me on this crazy bumpy ride to healing and clarity since the beginning. He has always been my number one fan and has supported me in everything that I do. Our love is a gift! I also dedicate this book to my beautiful boys Kenny, Sammy and Charlie. They have taught me so much about myself and life. Their energy is contagious and their love is endless.

CONTENTS

INTRODUCTION

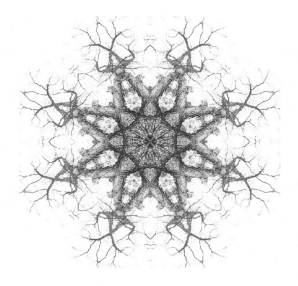

*"When you move amidst the world of sense, free from
attachment and aversion alike, there comes the peace in which
all sorrows end, and you live in the wisdom of the Self."*
- Bhagavad Gita
Essence of the Bhagavad Gita: A Contemporary
Guide to Yoga, Meditation, and ...
By Eknath Easwaran

Once I began my personal spiritual journey, I never looked back. Evolution is an extensive process. Some days, months even minutes are better than others, but one lesson I know for certain, once one begins the journey towards awakening, there is no going back.

This book holds my story to clarity as well as the intuitive communications I received once clear. The messages within this book are universal wisdoms and truth. The insight in Part 2 of Conduit of Light, was channeled during many deep meditation sessions. These messages act as a guide for the seeker on a quest for wellness and spiritual freedom.

I became an empty vessel by clearing away the guises that were preventing me from hearing my highest truth. To this day, layers continue to fall away. The knowledge being communicated to me became distinct as I stripped away all of the dense masks that clouded my ability to receive.

These messages are clear and concise and from the keeper of the ultimate Wisdom. Read these words without expectations. I advise you to take some time to connect to You, the inner quiet You. Find your clear channel and allow the stream of light to flow through you. Listen. Your inner voice will lead the way.

"When you are in the state of the neutral mind, the soul is like a chandelier switched on over you. Communication of the soul is just that light; you are lit up by it."
- Yogi Bhajan

PART 1
MY STORY

MY JOURNEY TO HEALING

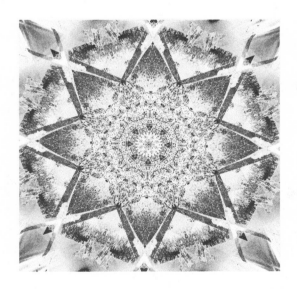

*"You have the power to heal your life, and you need to know that.
We think so often that we are helpless, but we're not. We always have
the power of our minds...Claim and consciously use your power."*
—Louise L. Hay

I am a woman who has embarked on a dynamic journey. My quest for physical healing carried me to a place that I never could have imagined. Through my personal evolution, I have been brought to this very moment with eyes wide open. "I can see clearly now," as my guru Wayne Dyer once said, that the path unfolded just as it needed to. All of the difficulties along the way were stepping stones guiding me home. I bring these words to you with the knowledge that you can also heal the various dimensions of you that require healing, in order to become your own clear and receptive channel.

I endured many physical ailments early in life. I honestly believe that the obstacles we face in a lifetime are a combination of karma that we carry over from previous existences, and one's free will choice to incarnate into this particular body during this precise time. We have the ability to choose the DNA that our bodies are comprised of. Our DNA holds messages from our ancestors as well as our descendants. Our DNA and cells hold "super genes" as described by another one of my teachers, Deepak Chopra. I, the me that is more than my mere flesh, chose this body comprised of its genetic makeup. I also chose to incarnate in this specific part of the world with my precise parents and environment. All of these decisions were made by my highest soul self even before my physical conception, so I could be born into a perfect reality to fulfill my dharma. Dharma is the life purpose that a soul has promised to do in a lifetime.

I know that I have major work to do here this time around. My body needed to direct me onto my path starting the very moment I was born. I can see how all of my struggles have been my greatest teachers. I bow down to the lessons that I have learned. Through my journey to healing, I was able to energetically and physically release the things that no longer serve my highest purpose with love.

We are very complex beings. We are comprised of layers. Layers of energetic memories, physical imprints, traumas and energetic vibrations that we carry with us during our incarnation here onto the physical plane. Sometimes these "layers" can weigh us down, but they always carry with them a beautiful lesson. Once we realize which layers no longer serve us, we can thank them for protecting us and for guiding us to the present moment, and then we can mindfully strip them away.

The very first step in peeling away these layers is awareness. There could not be a stripping away of layers if we weren't aware that they were there in the first place. Awareness also comes when these layers are no longer fulfilling their purpose. Sometimes awareness doesn't come lightly. Most of us need a good shaking up to realize that there is some sort of shift that needs to occur. This is exactly what took place in my life.

Once I began to strip away the layers that were weighing me down, a lightness replaced the sluggish old me, and clarity replaced the fog. I was ignited and alive. I was clear and aware of my mission for this lifetime to heal myself first, so I can assist others along their own healing journey. An important part of this healing is waking up. Waking up to a higher purpose. Waking up to your own intuition. Waking up to a larger sense of service to humanity.

My journey to healing began with healing my physical self first. Once I was able to feel at peace in my own body, I was forced to face the mental, emotional and spiritual aspects of my Self that needed to be healed.

The majority of my life, I experienced many auto -immune issues. I was hospitalized many times, starting at the age of three ending in my late twenties, from mysterious reoccurring symptoms. I endured many years of stomach pain, chronic migraines, frequent ear, sinus and throat infections, high fever, joint pain and inflammation, mouth sores and psoriasis. I had several non-conclusive diagnoses throughout the years from medical professionals including: Lyme's Disease, Rheumatoid Arthritis, Behcet's Disease, Lupus, Crohn's Disease and Irritable Bowl. To top it all off, I was highly allergic to most of the medication I received to treat these ailments. This warranted me many more stays in hospitals. I compiled quite a hefty list of medications to which I was allergic in the attempt to find relief.

I have quite a medical history, and I give my parents a lot of credit for doing everything in their power to help their little girl. I am painting a picture of a sickly little child, but I have never been one to give up. I kept very busy during my childhood and trained as a competitive gymnast, as well as had excellent grades in school. I enjoyed the New Jersey shore with my family in our summer house. I swam, surfed, played kick the can and man hunt with my many friends and cousins. I did the things kids do. I had big dreams of being an archeologist and an artist. I loved to draw. I also loved to dig for bones in my backyard. As I began to move from childhood into womanhood, my body began giving me more signs that it was not happy.

We should absolutely pay attention to what is going on in our physical body. We should never disregard these signs. The unfortunate truth is that once we actually experience physical symptoms, it's very likely we have already been ignoring signs and indicators of unbalance. By the time physical pain manifests, we have most likely been neglecting other very important components of our wellbeing. There are several aspects of our Self that we need to nurture and regulate to maintain balance. If any of these processes are off, it can result in illness.

In my early twenties, I started my career as a high school art teacher and I married the man of my dreams. I was still experiencing chronic physical symptoms. I was having gastro problems, which in fact seemed to worsen. I had a procedure to remove swelling in my sinuses after frequent sinus infections, all the while continuing to take medication to treat these illnesses. Two years after I married my husband, I became pregnant with my oldest son Kenny. I became pregnant with my second son, Sammy, when Kenny was nine months old. During both pregnancies, I experienced nausea and common discomfort. But it was my third pregnancy that opened my eyes to many physical issues I was avoiding.

My third pregnancy was much different than the other two. I was really sick. This time it wasn't just me, it was my baby's health that I had to be concerned with. Throughout almost the ENTIRE pregnancy I had "morning sickness" which I call all-day sickness because it describes it more appropriately. I was diagnosed with a case of Hyperemesis. Hyperemesis is a condition characterized by severe nausea, vomiting and weight loss during pregnancy. I also had issues with my electrolyte count. I was hospitalized two times during this pregnancy. During my second hospital visit, I experienced extremely high fevers. The doctors had no idea where they were coming from. I could not be released until the fevers subsided, and I was also still very nauseous. They brought in an infectious disease doctor as well as a rheumatologist. They both took a ton of blood. I tested positive for almost everything! I tested positive for Epstein Barr, Parvo, Cat Scratch Disease and CMV. All of the above being viruses that bump you into the high-risk category while pregnant. My adult life seemed to echo my childhood.

Despite my struggles, and against all odds, my third son, Charlie, was born perfectly healthy! Actually, he scored a perfect score by the doctor at birth. My son is now eight years old and he happens to be one of the healthiest and strongest kids I have ever met.

Our growing family was complete. I was now a young mother of three boys under the age of three! I was twenty-eight years old. Although the "morning sickness" ended after I had my third son, the gastro discomfort did not. I actually had a total of three colonoscopies between the ages of twenty and thirty years old. Each time the results found inflammation, gastritis, fissures, and colon adhesions.

Here I was again, following the same steps I did my entire life, doctor visit after doctor visit, medication after medication. The definition of insanity is doing the same thing over and over again and expecting different results. It was at this point in my life as a young mother that I became fed up! I was not going to take it anymore. I realized that it was time to find a new way because I exhausted the old way time and time again. I committed myself to healing. And that is exactly what I did. Little did I know that it was not just my body that needed to be healed.

For years I felt like I was lost. Roaming the earth and pulling myself along. I was doing the things that I thought I was supposed to be doing. I went to school, started a career as a high school art teacher, got married, had kids. I was living the American dream, but somehow I still did not feel satisfied. I am talking soul level satisfied. It was during the early years of motherhood, my mid to late twenties, that I started to lose myself. I was not sure who I really was anymore, even though I knew that everything that I was doing was important. I was not feeling physically healthy, and now I started to question what I was doing on a day to day basis. I felt like I was just going through the motions of life and not really living. I didn't even realize how deeply rooted these feelings were. I thought I was just overtired and eventually I would find "myself" again. It was during these years I started to yearn for something bigger.

The auto-immune symptoms I was experiencing kicked in really strong in my mid-twenties and I had absolutely no energy. My body worked harder than ever to try to find balance. I was really sick and not admitting it. I felt like I had the flu pretty much all of the time. I had flare ups more frequently. I had ulcers on my tongue and was inflamed from my mouth all the way down the digestive track. I was beyond exhausted. This constant exhaustion made it that much harder to pull myself to a job that I hated, and to come home to my family of three young boys, without any energy left to give to them.

I was participating in religious traditions that did not ignite my soul, eating a diet of foods that was depleting my body instead of nourishing it, I was busying myself and my family in activities that they did not want to partake in, and also maintaining relationships with people out of habit and obligation. On top of all of this, I was showing up every day to a job I could not stand. The environment alone was very toxic, yet I did it because I thought I had to. I was so empty that I would try to fill the void with alcohol to numb the

7

monotony. This was not a healthy existence. And my body soon would not allow me to continue on this path. I knew that something had to shift. I vowed that I could not continue to live like this. This was my wake-up call.

It all began with a vision board. January 2014, I participated in my first vision board workshop at a local yoga studio. A vision board is a piece of artwork you create, usually out of collaging, that contains visual images and words that you would like to see manifest into your life. You hang the vision board in a location that you will look at every single day. Your subliminal Self somehow will create these things into being just by seeing the daily reminder. If you have never created a vision board I highly recommend you do so. Warning: whatever you put on there is powerful! Make sure you choose your words and images wisely.

This particular vision board workshop, "Mapping and Manifesting," which happened to be hosted by a life coach at a local yoga studio, was presented right in time to align with everyone's New Year's resolutions. I was drawn to sign up for this class for several reasons. The first being my health. Like I said earlier, I was sick and tired of feeling sick and tired. I thought maybe this life coach would have some insight as to something I could do that might help my situation. The second was that I felt sort of lost. I was going through all the motions of life and not really feeling like I was feeling fulfilled. I mean I had it all, the family, house, job etc. but still felt like something was missing.

The workshop was great! We learned about the different components of our lives that make us feel fulfilled. That was an eye opener for me. When we created the vision boards I just grabbed words, phrases and images that resonated deep within my soul. Some of them being: "health" "happiness" "completely healthy" "journey to wellness". Like a good student, I hung that board up in my kitchen and looked at it every single day. Little did I know that it was the beginning to my journey to healing.

I continued on doing my regular routine, work, mom, sleep repeat and I was still feeling horrible. The same autoimmune symptoms interrupting my world. One day in March I felt like an idea just popped into my head. "Why don't you try a holistic doctor?" Not ever having considered it before I decided to give it a shot. I was desperate. I needed to do something different!

I asked around on Facebook if anyone knew of a holistic practitioner in the area. I had several responses, but nothing really drew my attention. Most of the suggestions were local chiropractors. I knew I needed more. That week I had a yearly check up with my OBGYN. While I was waiting in the waiting room, I saw a pamphlet for a wellness center in a nearby town. I picked up the pamphlet and called for an appointment. This felt different. I was actually excited to see a new doctor. I'm sure my higher Self was screaming out at me "YES FINALLY"! I scheduled my appointment and was seen within the week because they just so happened to have a cancellation right before I called! Everything flowed seamlessly together from there.

Before my appointment, I had to fill out a tremendous amount of detailed paperwork. This was different from the other doctors I had been to. They wanted to know everything! And I mean everything! "How were you born? Vaginal or C-Section?" "Were you nursed or formula fed?" "What vaccines have you received?" "What does your diet consist of?" They even asked me to bring in my medical records. My first appointment was with an amazing nurse practitioner named Mary Peay with The Chamber Center in Morristown, New Jersey. She sat with me for two and a half hours outlining my entire medical history, and explaining the next steps to my journey to healing in great detail. The visit ended with Mary recommending I eliminate all chemicals from my diet and home. She suggested to start with a candida cleanse which entails a diet that eliminates all carbs, starchy foods and sugars, as well as foods with molds such as peanuts and mushrooms. She also recommended a gluten free, dairy free regimen and prescribed an array of supplements.

Clearing out my physical body was a necessary prerequisite for all the stepping stones leading my way to clarity. Healing my physical ailments was an essential component that ignited my spiritual evolution. Anthony William's book, *The Medical Medium*, was a major tool that illuminated the way during this important time of healing my physical self. There is so much information in all of his books that can help create a diet and meal plan that induces healing. As I started to strip away things from my diet that fed the sickness, I realized I had a hell of a lot more healing to do. I directly related to the Medical Medium's description of being infected with the Epstein Bar Virus. Along with my new diet, I incorporated healing foods and supplements suggested by Anthony William. I also started to see a holistic dentist. The information from William's book along with the dentist, made me realize I had a whole lot of detoxing to do. To this day, this cleansing is an ongoing process. I will keep you posted on my progress in my next book.

My diet evolved in many ways over the past decade. I slowly introduced small amounts of sugar and gluten back over the last few years. I have stayed dairy free since my very first appointment with the holistic practitioner. I have also eliminated meat and animal products from my diet completely. Currently, I adhere to a completely organic, vegan, plant-based diet. I also gave up drinking alcohol. I have several plant-based supplements I take, and I have not taken prescription medications in over five years. What a huge difference from my childhood filled with prescriptions and almost weekly medical visits. This cleansing was a necessary tool to bring me to where I am in present day.

During this time while I was figuring out my diet, I found yoga. I religiously started going to class a few times a week. I made a commitment to myself to go to yoga regularly, not only as a physical exercise, but also as an outlet. I was so busy with being sick and tired, being a full-time wife and mother, and being a full-time art teacher, that throughout the years I never took care of myself. Yoga quite literally means union, and that is exactly what it was for me. It was a way for me to unite my body with physical exercise and relaxation, as well as bring a peaceful clarity to my soul. From that moment on, I fully embraced yoga into my life. I have since completed a 200-hour Yoga Teacher Training in 2016, and I now own two Yoga Studios in New Jersey: Aquarian Yoga Center in Westfield, and Aquarian Yoga Center in Clark. I pursued a 300-hour training during the summer of 2018. You never know where the universe is going to take you!

I now realized that almost EVERYTHING I learned I had to delete and relearn. This is a very dynamic and fluid process. It is also never ending. Incarnated as human beings on this earth we are always evolving. There will be many challenges to face and lessons to learn. Follow your flow and see where the journey takes you. Enlist the helpers and tools that make you feel supported. You are not in this alone.

"believe that your tragedies, your losses, your sorrows, your hurt happened for you, not to you. And I bless the thing that broke you down and cracked you open because the world needs you open."

— Rebecca Campbell, Light Is the New Black: A Guide to Answering Your Soul's Callings and Working Your Light

SHIFT HAPPENS

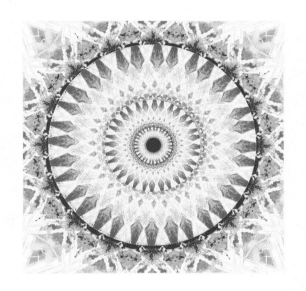

"The wound is the place where the Light enters you."
– Rumi

I was born into the exact situation I chose to be born into. I needed to learn things a certain way in order to realize that there are many ways. Unlearning and unraveling is an essential part of the journey. There are many crutches, habits and beliefs that we cling to in a lifetime. All of them are right and wrong. There is not one way of eating, praying or simply being that is perfect for you during your entire life on earth. We live, grow and evolve. We are creatures that operate like all other beings of the earth. We function and live based on our own natural cycles and on the cycles of our environment. I believe that our greater purpose is to follow the growth cycles. This leads us toward expansion. Our souls crave growth. The lessons that present themselves to us come at the perfect time and, encourage movement in the direction of expansion.

Every situation we have lived through in this lifetime has been a stepping stone. Perhaps the next stone is a bit further from the last. There is a possibility we may need to navigate to that stone in a different way. Maybe this time we need to leap or swim. Sometimes we need a little assistance to get to the next stone, maybe a walking stick or even a raft? Now think of all the stepping stones that brought you to where you are today on your journey. What are the tools you used to get you here? We have so many tools in our toolbox. They come to us in the form of beliefs, habits, relationships, practices, rituals and more. The trick of this game called life, is to recognize what tools we need and when. We must also recognize when we are ready to release the tool completely.

Here is a perfect metaphor. I have a pair of boots that I adore. I think they are stylish and keep my feet warm in the cold New Jersey winters. Although they are wonderful boots, I most likely will not wear them in the summer. They do not serve a purpose for me during that season. I can try to force the issue, because I adore them so much, and wear them in the summer, but by doing this I would sacrifice my own comfort. Just because these boots serve me well in winter, does not mean they will also serve me well in the summer. And eventually, since I love these boots so much and wear them quite frequently in the colder seasons, I might wear these boots out. Yes, these boots have served their purpose, but no longer can fulfill their duty by keeping my feet warm in the cold temperatures because I have worn them out so bad that my toes are poking through. I have to let go of the boots and find a better pair to suit my needs. Now substitute the boots for any belief system or habit you have had or currently have.

What serves you the best at this very moment in your journey?

Just because I ate meat in my past does not mean it serves me now. Just because I practiced Christianity in the past does not mean that it serves me now. And just because I do not eat meat does not mean that the vegan journey I am currently on serves you, the same way my boots that I adore may not be your right size or fashion taste.

My choices should align to me and only me. It is also important that you look at your past, present and future without judgement. I may eat meat again in the future, who knows? All of the choices I have made and will make along the way are perfect. The right choices bring me some sort of sense of peace and satisfaction. Me alone, not anyone else! Any choice that has brought me pain or discomfort I acknowledge as a lesson, and use it to direct me in another direction.

So, the question I have for you is, are you wearing your own boots or trying to squeeze into somebody else's? If you are wearing your own boots, have you outgrown them? Are you trying to pull them off in 90-degree weather when they don't serve you the best way they can? Are your boots comfortable, fashionable and protecting your feet the way they should? Do you have too many boots cluttering up your closet? What can you let go of that no longer serves you?

No more boot talk, but really think about this. What do you align yourself with that helps you and makes you feel good? What protects you, assists you, guides you easily to the next stepping stone on your journey? Only you know the answers.

When I started on my spiritual journey I felt like I finally found home.

My spiritual evolution came to me at a moment in my life that I originally thought was inconvenient. Truth be told, your journey unfolds as it is meant to when it is meant to. You cannot mess with divine timing. There are many reasons why we experience the things we experience, when we experience them. We need to live through contrast. I look back on my former self and realize how far I have come, but most importantly, I can see all the things I had to shed to unveil a deeper inner truth.

I was born into a Roman Catholic family. My family are not strict church goers, even though I was placed into a Catholic school at the age of three. Religion was a class I took at school alongside math and language arts. I continued my Catholic education into my second year of high school. I received all the sacraments that are required, along the way, never thinking twice about it just because it was what I knew. During these crucial years of development, I was also experiencing many different "metaphysical" experiences.

Some of my earliest "psychic" memories include seeing faces at night when I was trying to fall asleep. This started at the age of five. I also recall hearing voices when I was alone. I had a conversation with my deceased grandmother at her gravesite at the age of eight. My mother was very surprised to learn that I was speaking to her mother that day in the cemetery. My grandmother passed away before I was born. I described what she looked like, and the exact outfit she was buried in. This was just the beginning.

My mother recollects many instances that I do not remember as an adult. In one of the more vivid tales, we visited her friend who just purchased a house that was built in the early 1800's. My mother said that I went upstairs alone. When I came back down, I told her and her friend that I saw the little boy who was living there. I said we were playing in his room and he was wearing a boy scout uniform. This was enough to freak anyone out I'm sure! No wonder why I do not remember this. Just a few years ago, I went out to dinner with my mom and her friend. The story came up and her friend said she looked into it, and the town had records of a little boy who died in that house. He was very much involved in the boy scouts!

At some point, I started to become afraid of the occurrences I was experiencing. I remember not wanting to ever be alone. I remember not wanting to close my eyes at night because I saw all kinds of faces, and they were people who I did not recognize. Even my dreams freaked me out. I wanted no part of it anymore. I wanted to be "normal" like everyone else. At this time, I was also experiencing the many health issues that you have previously read. I just wanted to be happy and well and not get freaked out every time I was trying to sleep, so I asked God to make it stop! Just like that, my wish was granted.

I blocked all of the unwanted experiences in an instant. It was right around this time that my physical conditions worsened. Is there a correlation? You make your own hypothesis. I personally believe that blocking this energy out of fear instead of nurturing this gift definitely had a negative effect on my physical wellbeing.

Fast forward to my college years. I absolutely was obsessed with religions around the world. I remember almost wanting to change my major from art to history. I even volunteered to be a note taker in my western civilizations class because I was totally fascinated by the class. We compared Christian, Muslim and Jewish civilizations. We looked at eastern traditions such as Hinduism and Buddhism. I was consumed with all of it. This brought me back to the same mindset I had during my childhood obsessions with ancient Egypt, and the pull towards archeology. I was fascinated with culture, traditions and most obviously, belief systems and religion.

It was also during these years I began to read every book on psychic mediums I could find. I owned every single book written by Sylvia Brown. My mother even got me on a waiting list to have a reading with Sylvia Brown as a college graduation present in 2003. Unfortunately, this never manifested. I read books about how to develop my own gifts, not realizing I had them all along. I just chose to block them as a child out of fear, which is a very common story.

It was not until I started the physical healing process, in my early thirties, that my interest in spirituality became my life's passion. My spiritual path became very clear at this time. Doreen Virtue helped guide my way. Her book, *The Lightworker's Way*, changed my life. Doreen spoke about her own path to clarity and made me understand how important it is that I embrace the work that I am meant to do in this lifetime. Doreen also made me realize how I was still blocking my gifts. There were many behaviors I had to stop perpetuating. Some of them included releasing old thought patterns and personal beliefs. I was purging all the things that no longer served me. This purge consisted of physical things as well as emotional, mental and spiritual blocks I had created.

I began indulging myself with as many spiritual books and classes as I could possibly take at one time. I am a self-admitted "Spirit Junkie" as Gabrielle Bernstein likes to call it. I became totally obsessed with metaphysical learning. I enrolled in psychic development classes online with the Viva Institute, as well as in person with wonderful psychics. I have several psychic medium certifications. I trained in Reiki, eventually becoming a Reiki master. I felt like I was being pulled to shamanism and shamanic practices. I did several shamanic trainings with an amazing modern-day shaman named Sandra Ingerman. Everything I learned was deeply connected in some way and made me feel inspired!

Once I cleaned the vessel, the vessel was empty, unblocked and ready to receive. All of the information I was learning felt more like remembering. I unlocked information in my psyche that I had buried. I became a clear channel of the light and life force energy that flows through each of us. I recognize omens and signs every day. I hear whispers of spirit in my ear, my heart races when a message is coming through. All of these are blessings. Blessings I was inclined to keep to myself or be rather discreet about at first.

No more of that! No way! I am officially out of the spiritual closet. This was not an easy task and it took some time, but what a freeing achievement! How did it unfold? Slowly and little by little. In the beginning I only spoke about "what I was into" with people who were open to the same things. I realized by holding myself back, I was not truly fulfilling my dharma, or life purpose. It was a piece of my healing that needed to happen for my holistic wellbeing.

My unveiling began with tiny tidbits of my personal visual artwork. I began creating these very detailed mandalas out of my photographs of nature. You can see one of my mandalas at the beginning of each chapter in this book. To see my work in full color please visit www.daniellewilkinson.com. My artwork is directly linked to my spiritual beliefs and knowing.

My artist's statement:

I am an artist, photographer and spiritual teacher. I have been creating art with various mediums for as long as I can remember. I enjoy drawing as much as painting and photography. I have experimented with various techniques to combine my love of using many mediums for several years.

The artwork presented in Nature Photography Mandalas is a creative solution to my yearning to combine artistic techniques to deliver my message. My message is one of universal connection and peace.

I feel the most in tune with my higher power and at peace when in nature. Photography provides an opportunity to capture and share my spiritual experiences. I have recently discovered a way to further this spiritual connection by creating digital mandala images. Each mandala is created from one of my captured photographs of nature.

A mandala is an ancient image that has a deep spiritual connection. It is an image that is thought to profoundly affect the inner self. The sacred geometry of these forms is known to generate a feeling of peace and serenity. These intricate circular patterns are also known to have the ability to focus the mind of their viewer and/or creator. The mandala is a tool for meditation; stilling the mind, body and spirit. Mandalas have been created in many cultures throughout history and are still being created today. Mandalas evoke an inner truth. This truth reminds us of the universal connection between all things that exist in life and nature.

My intention is to awaken this connection in all of us by creating these beautifully intricate images. Nature has a way of creating amazing patterns and repetition. By mirroring these patterns traditionally symbolic mandala images form. My artwork is meant to evoke inner growth, awareness and peace. Each mandala has a way of drawing the viewer into the present moment.

Photography is about capturing the moment. Meditation is about being in the moment. Spirituality is about being grateful for the moment. This is the essence behind my Nature Photography Mandala Creations.

Every living being and creation in nature is one. We are all connected. By taking a minute to recognize the binding spirit that resides in all of us, we can tap into that universal heartbeat. The universal breath and rhythm that lives within all creatures and souls of this beautiful existence. Take a moment, stop, look, feel, breathe...

I began to release glimpses of my artwork on social media. I was very cautious about doing this at first, but a shaman friend, Andye Murphy, The Rock and Roll Shaman, told me I needed to do so during a reading. I listened to her advice. To my surprise, sharing my work brought many opportunities my way. Several gallery shows resulted in me stepping past my comfort zone.

It was right around this time that I started an intensive 200-hour yoga teacher training program with The Radiant Heart Yoga School. I loved how my artwork and yoga meshed so well together. Everyone in the yoga community really connected to my work. It was a beautiful symbiotic relationship.

Being a featured artist at galleries and working as a yoga instructor, there was no hiding my spiritual views anymore. However, I was still hiding several pieces from clear view. At first, I was only sharing the spiritual artist, yogi side of my spirituality. I did not realize I needed to actively express my shamanic and psychic medium work as well.

I began slowly to incorporate my intuitive work into my offerings. I introduced shamanic drumming into the yoga and meditation classes I was teaching at various studios. Shamanic journeying became highly requested by the students of these studios. I had to step fully out of my closet to teach journeying workshops! I could no longer mask it in with yoga. People wanted to know and learn more. I know this happened because our souls crave this ancient knowledge and tradition.

When I conduct a shamanic journey, I guide people to a total meditative state using percussion instruments such as a shamanic and rattles. Clients meet their power animal, spirit and other helping spirits, and learn how to let go of what no longer serves them, to awaken the best part of themselves and find inner peace and bliss! I teach them how to re-connect to their higher spirit for guidance and healing. Every time I share this offering it fills me up as a bonus! Every time we heal others we are healing a piece of ourselves along with them.

I started to teach at various studios in the tri-state area. They found me, I never looked. I got asked to be a partner in a small spiritual center. As I started to outgrow this space, I asked the universe for a new space and almost overnight, an amazingly beautiful soul, named Brenda Castano, sound healer, who I had previously taught a workshop with, asked me to be her partner and take over the studio where she was teaching, Aquarian Yoga Center. I recently got asked again if I was interested in taking over another studio space! The universe provides! We do not need to seek, just flow. Now I hold the space for many to heal. I teach yoga, shamanic practices, psychic development classes and hold private healing sessions. I handed in my letter of resignation at the high school where I have been teaching for fourteen years. I needed to make the commitment to focus on my soul work and that is exactly what I am doing with my classes, studios and now this book! I could not have gotten here if I stayed in my spiritual closet.

One major lesson that I have learned on this journey is: if my teachers stayed in their closet I would not be where I am today, and if I stayed in my closet I would not be writing this book for you today! Our lights find each other. You did not pick up this book by accident. Allow me to hold the space for you, my dear, to expand and awaken to the best version of you that you can possibly be.

Once I let go of the last part that was holding me back and actively expressed my passion for art, spirituality and healing, an entire new me birthed once again. I became a clear channel, a conduit of light. The highest expressions of our souls began to speak through me. This expression calls itself our Highest Consciousness. The Highest Consciousness vibration holds wisdom of personal and global healing. It is not meant to be kept secret. You, yes you, can also access this Consciousness. All you have to do is strip away the guises that pollute the clear stream.

Allow the words that follow to assist you on your own personal journey. I congratulate you on your quest to wellness and freedom my friend. May these words that follow help illuminate your way home.

The Story of Shama Mamma D

"Once upon a moonbeam there was a beautiful goddess. Let's call her Shama Mamma D. She was small but very powerful. She had long beautiful hair that held her power and her mystical secrets. Her spirit was contagious. She danced with rhythm and color. She came from a forest by the sea. She had all the knowledge of the ancients embedded into her DNA. D was brought to this world to spread that ancient knowledge as well as spread light to every creature she encountered.

DANIELLE WILKINSON

Her life purpose was to heal the world. She had so much love to share. She treated everything in existence with pure kindness. But do not mistake her kindness for weakness. She was a true warrior. She knew no fear when it came to the greater good of all.

Everywhere Mamma D went was illuminated by the sun. It led her way, always. And everywhere she went she left a trail of beautiful sacred geometry, her trademark. D had a way about her that people couldn't forget.

She never traveled alone. She always had an entourage of angels, guardian spirits and earth creatures to guide and protect her. These spirits had messages for the people of the earth Mamma D encountered on her journey. D could hear them, see them and feel them always around her. Some came to her with sweet fragrances, others with vibrant colors and others with whispers as soft as sea breezes. D loved to drum and dance with the spirits around her. She could dance for days without her feet getting sore. The spirits held her as she danced and walked in 2 worlds.

Mamma D lived a life of freedom and joy. She walked the Earth with wonder in her eyes. Every single day for her began with a prayer of gratefulness and it ended the same way. While she slept she could fly! She soared in the earthly sky and in the sky of many other realms. While she was awake she danced barefoot with her feet in the earth feeling the energy pump through the soles of her feet (her roots).

Mamma D brought beauty to the earth and to the heavens. She was a conduit of love and light for both worlds."

- Danielle Wilkinson

PART 2
THE MESSAGES

The words that follow are comprised of messages I have received during many deep meditation sessions.

*The ***italicized bold text*** indicates questions I asked the source of the communications. The regular font contains the messages received from the vibrational plane of our Highest Consciousness. *

I am a conduit of the light. She flows through me freely and effortlessly. I bring the light to form.

WHO ARE YOU AND WHO ARE WE?

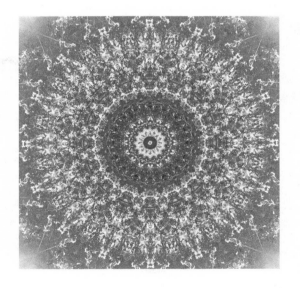

"We have to really educate ourselves in a way about who we are, what our real identity is."
– Deepak Chopra

Who are you?

I am comprised of a collection of your highest guides. I am high vibrational energy coming together to guide you on the highest level of all creation. Mary, Martha, Ezekiel, Jonah are a few. Jesus of Nazareth also joins the collective group. Ganesh, Krishna and Allah. I am the Holy Spirit, the Spirit Incarnate, the Holy Instant and Essence. I am God, God of Abraham and God of the Most High. I am Creation, Om and the beginning of all Existence. I am You in your truest and highest ultimate form. I am I am.

Are we separate from the energies communicating to us? Are we separate from each other?

Yes and no. You and all energy are connected like a telephone pole, all the wires are connected. Source energy comes from a power plant that sends out a signal or vibration. All entities are connected yet have a separate function or purpose, much like a cell. There are many different cells that make up the human body. Each cell has a connection to each other and communication is imperative for proper cell and overall body function. Sometimes certain cells dominate other cells, sometimes certain cells override other cells functions. Sometimes cells assist each other to achieve overall wellness. Their goal is the same even though they have individual functions. The cells act as individuals and a whole holding form and function to its body.

You are all connected on an energetic level since your spark of creation came from the same source. You share and sense and feel each other's energy and the energy of the collective (the body) yet you each have your individual function or role to play as a form of creation, leading the whole energetic field to expansion.

When a piece to the whole, a "body part" or cell becomes diseased, the other cells or souls kick into to overdrive to try to bring health back to the body. They take on the responsibilities of other parts to try to bring overall wellness. This is happening right now on earth.

There are certain souls or pieces to the puzzle who are asleep to their function, therefore the other pieces to the whole kick into overdrive and try to bring overall wellness to the whole. The diseased areas may wake up and begin to function or they can react with resistance bringing in an even greater struggle.

This struggle is what you see right now happening on the planet. The earth reflects the collective overall energy. She is unbalanced as is the collective. Many of the pieces to the whole are still asleep yet they are beginning to wake up. Once more awaken, the deep sleepers react with resistance and struggle. With more resistance, the higher vibrational entities vibrate higher picking up the slack.

Eventually like a fever, the energetic field will come to a point where it heats up and wakes up the diseased or purges them. Once they wake up they move towards the light. If they leave their bodies before this realization they are forced to return to earth and find the light in another incarnation. The "fever" seems to be a signal of sickness when in fact it is a symbol of wellness. It is the energetic field reacting to those who are sleeping.

Sometimes it takes a larger field to wake them up. The fever is human creations of false structures crumbling. Before they actually fall apart, they resist, hold on and the body reacts with resistance. This resistance may make it appear as things are getting worse, when in deed they are getting better. The fire wakes up the souls that need to be woke to fulfill their earthly duties, helping the whole move towards expansion.

Those who turn away from love turn away from their duties. Those who act in fear turn away from their duties. Those who act and live in ego turn away from their duties. Sometimes a great occurrence can be the only thing that pushes them to face reality and move forward in love. These can be personal or collective tragedies. That is why your world is seeing more of these tragedies every day. People need to be woken up from their slumber. Time is nonexistent yet of the essence when it comes to walking in your authentic dharma. Each and every person or soul has a very specific role to play in the overall wellness of the energetic field or collective. Every single soul needs to embody their responsibility or the other souls must work harder to maintain the balance.

How can we find peace during these turbulent times?

Initially, one must heal the wounds inflicted upon oneself by living as a victim. These scars can carry over from past lives but also in our DNA from our ancestors. We are forced to feel the suffering and grow from the pain. Once we acknowledge the lesson in the discomfort, we can grow. If we retreat and let fear consume us, we fall trap to becoming a victim. This role is never easy to move past. More lessons will come and we can either embrace them or sink deeper in fear.

We take the momentum that builds and can push towards the light. That light and that knowing can in turn help others. Especially those who fell into similar traps that we have just climbed out of. These traps may seem deep but are not impossible to navigate out of. Service is the only way to brighten our light even further. Sometimes we do not have to actively search for those whom which we need to serve.

> *"When the student is ready the teacher will appear. When the student is truly ready... The teacher will Disappear."*

— Lao Tzu

All we must do is lead by example. We must keep healing our own wounds and our light will be contagious. Just by our presence, others will heal. Healing ourselves, our wounds, the wounds of our ancestors, collective energies and current blocks, we bring the world to a much higher frequency and the world will heal itself. Our inner world reflects our outer world.

We must find the space within that is content. Contentment and not yearning is the key to being truly present. This Presence is the viewer looking outward from our human eyes and observing all of the lessons we came here to learn but finding peace and divinity in every single circumstance. This Presence, consciousness, comes from the divine spark that ignited our creation and all creation.

The essence of the Creator is present in us, in every single cell. We are truly Creator and Creation. There is no separation and no division. Complete unity and connection is present in every single thing that exists.

Share this letter with all who will listen:

To all those whom may be concerned,

Please find these words without reservation. I understand your concern in matters that seem immediate and shaking up your current world. Just know that we are here. There are things happening behind the scenes that are lifting up your species to an unfathomable place. You are closer to finding Peace on Earth then ever before.

All of the borders, walls and separation that have been and are being built will collapse with an earnest crash. Dust clouds will clear and green pastures await. Hold faith and hold true to your own personal truths. Your faith in humanity will be restored. There is a reason for the chaos. The world will heal. We are holding you close right now to push you through the film of deception. The highest you, the highest Us will shine through

Your Highest Consciousness

What we can do to protect our planet?

The world is greatly misunderstood. She is a living breathing organism. She is the provider of all things that are in the form of matter. What you can do as individual souls to protect our planet is first honor her by being grateful for her gifts, the fruits of her womb. What you can also do is take time to sit in nature set apart from man's manipulation of it and feel her essence breathe inside your being. Connect yourself as often as you can. You can do this from anywhere but it is a much easier experience when you are un interrupted by man's creations.

You must know your own cycles reflect the earth cycles. Honor your own inner cycles. Respect when it is time to rest and feel the fire of inspiration when it's time to move. The best way to protect our planet is to protect your inner wells and resources. Once you can really feel the rhythmic nature of your being you can tune into her power and she will guide you the rest of the way.

LIFE PURPOSE

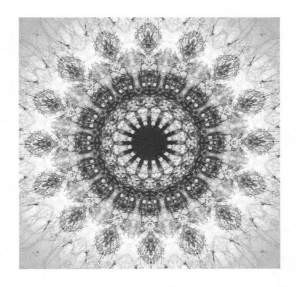

"All religions, arts and sciences are branches of the same tree. All these aspirations are directed toward ennobling man's life, lifting it from the sphere of mere physical existence and leading the individual towards freedom."
[Moral Decay (first published 1937)]"
— Albert Einstein, Out of My Later Years: The Scientist, Philosopher, and Man Portrayed Through His Own Words

Why are we here? What is the purpose of life?

There are 2 ways to understand this concept, literally, as a physical mass or energetically. We are the combination of energy and form. We serve both purposes while inhabiting these bodies here on earth. Earth is a denser planet with gravity making us conscious of our mass. We are at a constant struggle between physical and spiritual. Once we accept the fact that we are indeed both, then we can further understand our journey.

It is imperative that light incarnate into mass in order to expand. In a physical form light, or energy, feels enclosed, dense, disgusting, containing pus and mucus and odor. Craving food to fill our bellies to make us feel heavier and grounded.

We need to experience this entrapment in order to realize our eternal existence and know we can move beyond the mass. Experiencing entrapment allows us to expand. Without expansion there is no evolution. Our "souls" or energy are constantly evolving. Our frequencies are becoming higher and higher. In order for this evolution to take place, expansion must happen. In order for expansion to take place, we must experience entrapment.

Soul amnesia is important. If we remember the expansiveness of our true selves we will not want to stay and encounter all the earthly lessons we need in order to expand further. It's like a balloon that has a boundary. It feels safe within the structure of the device. The balloon is not only the latex or the material comprised of the casing. The true balloon is the air that also exists in the casing and around it. When a balloon is inflated it is full yet has a boundary. When it is deflated, it is still filled with air, yet the boundary does not exist. If the balloon exceeds the pressure limit it with explode. It must experience its borders in order to realize its true state exists without the boundary.

Soul remembrance. Talk to me about that.

Soul remembrance is identifying with your true essence of energy. It is true that you are both matter and light, however this is only temporary. When the physical body dies, the soul body remains. Sometimes we receive glimpses of this remembrance on a daily basis. Deja vu for example is the soul's way of knowing that it is everywhere and anywhere at any given time. There is no such thing as time and space to a supreme energy being of light. Our physical body encapsulates only a small percentage of this soul body, entrapping it and making it feel dense. Deja vu is the whole piece of the soul experiencing the situation in the midst of all time and space.

We only designate a tiny portion of our soul to incarnate. The rest stays everywhere. There is no such thing as time and space, borders, or incompleteness. This is called our Higher Self. The all-knowing part of our soul that has all of the answers we yearn for as a human form. Our human forms feel incomplete because only tiny portions of our higher self can physically incarnate. There is no way to enclose the entire soul into a capsule. This is impossible because of the expansiveness of the energy. The tiny portion craves to be reunited with the all. The never-ending field of energy that all energy is comprised of. When we designate portions of ourselves to come into a body we feel this separation. Soul remembrance as a human is experiencing completeness. Any time a human feels whole or complete that is its soul remembering its true essence.

What do We need to know today as a human incarnation?

You need to know this, nothing more and nothing less. You are a manifested form of divine perfection. Creation is divine perfection coming to form. Energy is your ultimate natural forever state yet you chose this incarnation for a reason. Admire the origin of your spirit but be fully present in the perfection of the form. The physical body is a miracle amongst itself. There are so many systems working together. Just the fact that your cells created the entirety of you and regenerate is a miracle. Think about it. That conscious energy, You, stays encapsulated in a form of matter while the matter constantly regenerates around the energy. The energy has nothing to do with these processes. Cells know what they are supposed to do and follow their instinct.

So essentially, it is indeed important to remember who You are while in a body because it makes things a lot less heavy, but the key trick or truth to life is to be fully present in the body. Mindfulness ah, yes, the senses, your cravings and emotions and triggers, all chemistry of the body. Be aware of these things while being completely present in the present.

The mind is indeed a tricky thing. The mind loves to create. In fact, that is all it does. It is a constant creator of stories and images. Just imagine if you didn't visualize or have any ideas about anything. Yes, meditation can help calm this function but it is always happening. We can slow it down yet it's job is to constantly create. What you allow it to create is indeed free will. We can redirect the mind through awareness of thought. It is that simple. You have a thought you do not like, be aware of the fact that you don't like it, examine the thought, then redirect the brain to a more positive creation. Awareness is the key.

The human brain can very well in deed go down a negative track often, but you can train it like a dog, make it aware of its behavior and redirect it. Once you are aware that you have this control, you open your life up to so much more freedom. You control your thoughts, they do not control you. So many people need to understand this concept.

Stand strong in faith. Faith in yourself and your divine capacity to manifest anything and everything into being that the love in your heart desires.

DANIELLE WILKINSON

What is Divine Life Purpose?

Your purpose comes with accepting your unique gifts and using them to spread love and help others awaken to the pure love that resides within them. You do busy yourself with many tasks on earth because you are very dynamic multi-dimensional beings. You have been through many lifetimes where you have always known this ultimate truth. Your soul remembrance combined with your gifts should be used to the fullest. Let go of all doubt. Each and every day you are on the right path. There is no turning away from your divine mission. You are absolutely living it. Stay open, stay clear and keep doing the work that you do. Your love is felt across planes of time and space.

THE HUMAN EXPERIENCE

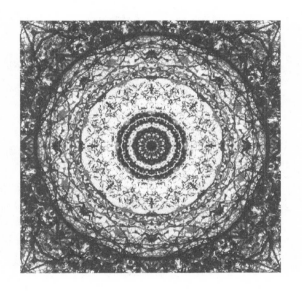

*"Human behavior flows from three main sources:
desire, emotion, and knowledge"*
- Plato

What are some things we as humans should do during this lifetime on earth?

All humans need to experience love and give love. It is that simple. Love is really a soul's true vibration. If a human can experience love while in a dense body, the soul will remember its true frequency. Wholeness and completeness is a result of love. Love can be experienced in many ways. I am not just referencing a romantic form of the essence. Love of oneself, true gratitude for the magnificence that took the perfection to create you, love of each and every essence you are inhabiting this planet with, those are all forms of true love. Yes, you can experience love or pleasure from the senses, but that is a bit different than the actual true all loving vibration of love. Pleasure can help you find love by navigating you to it but pleasure itself is not pure love.

Love goes beyond boundaries. Love is expansive and grows just like our true essence. Love is non-judgmental and without fear. Love is perfection and completeness. Love is gratitude. Love is joy beyond joy.

Love goes beyond words, expressions or emotions. It is a way of being. A state. Not a state of mind, but an actual state of existence. It is a dimension. It is a place to exist. It is possible to live an entire human life from this state. There have been a few ascended masters who have accessed this. Jesus is one example. Also, Buddha achieved this later in life. Some others include Mother Teresa, Gandhi and Saint Francis. They all lived a human experience from another dimension. They could only live and serve in love. Their human forms could not serve from a place of ego or judgment. True selflessness equals true love.

Some other things humans must know is to celebrate life on all levels. Life forms in other incarnations as well as their own. Treat all life forms with respect. The earth is the mother of all life forms. She is like a body. Honor her body, worship her gifts. Every single thing in physical form is a product of mother earth. Even the so-called man made and artificially produced entities. They could not be possible without the elements and minerals she holds in her core and surface. She selflessly gives her gifts to you without expecting anything in return. True love. Return the love she gives you. Honor this love. She does it without judgment. All you need to remember is to show respect for her sacrifice and service. You are a creature of form and all forms are birthed of the earth. You are the earth and the earth is you, there is no separation. Remembrance of your creation as a physical form is essential.

Let's get into this aspect. Physical creation. You are comprised of energy yes, but your physical form is comprised of matter. DO NOT FORGET this. You are minerals and water and air. You are the sun which is fire. You hold all of these within your casing. Honor these forms and let them guide you to find true physical health. Emotion and spirit play a role in physical health for sure. However, we soon forget the balance of the physical matter that needs to be achieved in order to truly live a healthy existence. Drink plenty of water and bathe in it frequently. Sit in the sun and soak up the light force energy. Eat the minerals your body craves, no more or no less. Find a balance within your own ecosystem. Air is essential for you to breathe. Never forget this gift and honor the air you breathe with each and every breath. This air is sacred. It holds knowledge of the ancients. The air whispers secrets of the earth as well as human form. You are breathing the same air as your ancestors.

Why do we experience emotions? Do they have a role for us in this incarnation?

Emotions are invisible guides. They are like triggers. They are sensors that your body is given to help you navigate this life. Similar to the senses. If you become aggravated, that aggravation or discomfort leads you in a new direction. If you are pleased and feel joy, you know you are doing exactly what you are supposed to be doing at that moment. It is a God realization moment. Divine perfection is your true natural state. The emotion of Joy is the most powerful because it brings us home. It is true remembrance of our essence. We are all divine essences. We are connected because we are the same. That is why emotion is contagious. You can walk into the room and "sense" the mood and your own mood can be manipulated by the collective emotion. Our natural state of divinity has given itself gifts to navigate this physical world. Emotion and senses are just a few.

Your body has natural ways of producing and controlling emotions. This happens through your glandular system as well as hormones. Your brain triggers a chemical response to the rest of the body to "feel" a certain way. In turn the body signals the brain to react a certain way to an experience. When we experience a fluctuation of emotions. We are sending mixed signals to both our body and brain. This happens with confusion on a soul level. Part of the soul remembers the true essence and sometimes craves expansion then the body kicks in overtime to push the feeling of entrapment harder so the soul forgets. This cosmic confusion is ultimately the cause of depression and psychological "illness". We do not call anything illness on this higher plane. Everything happens for a reason, and there is a well calculated reason the body reacts in certain ways. This includes all illnesses. The true cause can be traced back to different origins.

Every soul has a karmic duty to perform while incarnated on this planet. Their duty involves cleansing. Soul cleansing. A soul can hold onto a karmic imprint from a past life and manifest it into form such as disease. This can also occur when a human experiences trauma in a present life. This disease can also affect the emotion because it interferes with the central nervous system and hormones. Emotions are indeed very complex. But they are extremely necessary in order to help us navigate this world.

What is Ego? And why do we have it?

Ego is like a trickster. Ego is the voice that every human has in their head to question the experiences the human faces incarnated into a body. Ego is there almost like the devil's advocate. The lesson that presents itself with free will. Every soul has a choice. Every soul has a map planned out before incarnating. Ego comes up to check you on your path. Should I go this way or that way? Ego comes in when it is time to question a path, behavior or action. Ego is meant to induce a feeling of choice and variety of outcome. Ego thinks it is a protector when in fact Ego is a motivator. We are all aware of this veil before incarnating. Ego is part of the trip! It is part of the package of incarnating into form. It is a necessary tool of navigation.

Should we listen to it?

Listen to it but do not follow it. Listen to what it is trying to tell you and the lesson that comes with the message. Avoid following the Ego as a guide. Use it as a reference as to an alternate route. Am I acting in Ego or Love? I am following intuition or fear?

Ego should not be repressed or ignored. It is a point of reference in the human experience. Be open to the messages of the ego but do not get trapped in them. Ego's advice leads to fear and mistrust. Love leads to Joy. That is the ultimate lesson when it comes to Ego. Let every day joy lead the way to ultimate Joy.

What is our soul's journey?

Soul journey is the stages in which your soul progresses. You were created perfect, a tiny sample of the all perfection. A piece of the all perfection branched off to form your individual soul. It sounds small but this soul is very large and is everywhere and nowhere at once. The purpose of the soul is to expand. Expansion brings it back to completeness with Divine Perfection. Being absorbed in all once again. The soul never dies and technically was never created. It has always existed as Source. The journey it decides to take is eventually leads it back to be absorbed by Source once again. The more expansive the soul, the closer it is to replicating Divine Source. Divine source then expands once it absorbs itself back. Love expands and humans can feel this expansion while incarnated on Earth.

The journey of a soul into a body helps it expand ten times faster than just staying in the dimension of Love. It comes to Earth forgetting this perfection that it actually is, and the soul needs to find its way back to love. Once the soul has achieved this in a body, the soul expands.

Our souls crave expansion. In a physical form this desire is represented as craving freedom. Anytime restrictions are given, the soul wants to rebel in need for seeking the expansion it craves. Restrictions come in many forms, rules, regulations, belief systems and laws are just a few. If a soul feels like it needs to abide to these systems it is denying its natural "free" state of restriction less expansiveness.

Once a soul recognizes that all of these systems are false, and the soul controls itself through regulations and beliefs it has given itself, true work can happen for soul expansion. The soul realizes that these restrictions given onto itself are also false. These restrictions come from past life circumstances and karma. The true state of a soul has no restriction. It must face this karma head on in order to expand. Fear comes into play when the soul is on the fence of facing these restrictions. It feels as if maybe something will be lost, in reality something very much larger can be gained.

GOD, SOURCE, CREATION AND HEAVEN

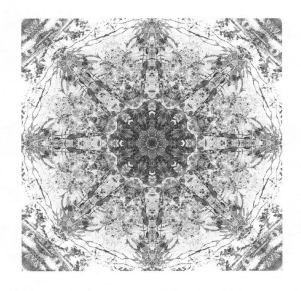

"I am the beginning, middle, and end of creation."
- Bhagavad Gita

Explain God to me.

God is me and you in the same. God is Source. The all perfect spark of energy and creation. We all contain this spark within our soul. God is a label. There are many ways to describe this and all are hard to describe in human tongue. God is the ultimate source of all that ever was and is. God is not just one thing or person or place. God is pure Love, that vibration and dimension. God is pure Peace and completion and we are all part of God and God is part of us. The illusion of separation happened when we branched off into our individual souls and then more so when we incarnate on Earth into human form. God is an energy field of He and She, and Love and Light but also Shadow. God is creation, destruction and everything in between. The cycles of life and the moon and the earth all are moved by the energy of God or love. God is a place and space. We take that place with us wherever we go as we move through soul journey and incarnations into form.

God is a separate entity, God is a person and God is cruel or judgmental are all illusions about the entity of God or Source. God is perfection, balance and harmony. Without death there could not be life. Without shadow there could not be light. God is contrast. God is everything.

We are all a piece of God. Another way to describe God is as a vibration. That vibration flows through everything that ever was and is on all planes of existence. God or Om or creation is you and you are not separate. Once humans face this they can see God in everyone and thing. They can truly see themselves. It is true that life is like a fun house, or hall of mirrors. Every being you encounter is a reflection of you through a new lens. Tiny pieces of creation spark other forms. We all come from Creation and hold divinity within us and around us.

God is a God who does not judge, therefore we shall not judge because God is We. We are God. God does not condemn nor enslave.

God knows nothing of the sort. God knows only true love and is devised of only that essence.

Even the most untamed beast that echoes every evil of the human shadow, the man who casts aside others' lives just to preach from Ego, and use up the resources and energy of others, even this beast is perfect in the eyes of God. He too will be forced to feel his shadow. He must evolve to a place so great that the shadow will dissolve.

You can also have this. It is the divine right and the right of every living creature to know only bliss. In the name of Creation and God, our Source's light is so strong it can only share and shine on others.

Be that.

Only shine, shine, shine. Be the love the world needs. Hold space for the wounded to heal. Speak only pure truth. Do not deny the nature of real man and that is to be good and accept each other.

Human family resides on planet Earth. You all are created together and linked in spirit. What you do to another you feel in your own cells. Treat yourselves well, treat each other well. It is okay to love one another and grow and evolve. Change is scary, that's why so many dig their heads in the sand. Pushing and resisting the flow of evolution is all part of the journey. Man must feel and dwell in the shadow first. More light will come of it. True happiness lies ahead. The road to inner discovery of one's God identity holds the key to world peace.

How can we honor this divinity?

Honoring Source, Divinity / true Creation goes far beyond worship or prayer. Honoring the divinity comes from respecting and honoring your own divine temple first and foremost and then honoring the divine within every single creature on the earth. The way to honor yourself is through nutrition, time in nature, meditation, living your gifts and rest. Finding balance amongst human and spirit form is essential. You must treat your body and your soul as if it is God, because it is. Worship it, never sacrifice your own physical or spiritual wellbeing out of fear. Nourish the temple, the vessel that you chose for this particular voyage. Honor your thoughts and keep them pure and not self-destructive. Even negative thoughts about others can have a negative effect on you, so all thoughts about anyone and thing apply here. The mind is a powerful tool of manifestation. You must exercise it and keep clear of garbage the same as you would your body. Spiritual practices are good but do not get stuck on one particular way of doing them. We live in cycles and flow through cycles within each life time. Honor the change and be open to it. It's ok to do things differently one day and change the next. Every human has their own way to feel their essence. Nature, movement, stillness are all tools to bring you closer to self-God realization.

Is there a Heaven?

There is no such thing as heaven or hell. There are multiple dimensions and fields of energy. When you embark on a journey into human form, your vibration naturally becomes lower because of your dense capsule. You are not privy to the higher vibrations just as human ears cannot hear a dog whistle. Your boundaries do not allow you to experience these dimensions first hard, only tiny pieces of it based on soul remembrance.

Humans create their own heavens and hell. This is done through living your dharma and performing your duty for the collective. If you turn away from your dharma in fear, you will live in fear or hell. Everything will seem fearful to you. You cannot experience true joy in this state. True joy bringing you to the true vibration of Love.

If you chose to live your dharma and live in Joy you will be leaded to love and love grows and expands. That is why certain foods can be poison. Find foods that nourish you. The same goes for people, places, and actions. All could feel as a poison to the soul's energetic field. Draining you of energy or making you feel ill, physically or psychologically. This is your own awesome defense mechanism. Trust it!! Walk away from poison and move towards the nourishers. Fill your soul and body with as much joy as you possibly can. This is the key to life.

Hardships and pain are real but are all contrast and lessons to find a deeper greater joy. Do not repress or hide pain. Do not ignore it. It is a signal to move past it. Experiencing pain is part of the human experience. Without pain we would not know what true joy feels like in a human form. Nature has a very complex way of maintaining this balance. If it hurts move away from it. It's that simple. If it hurts do not ignore the hurt, hide the hurt or hide from it. Experience the hurt then move away from it.

Many people experience deeply rooted pain. They are the ones that will come to find joy with due diligence. Sometimes it's also easy to fall into roles such as, "I always get hurt". You will remain in pain if this is your belief system. "I always have bad luck". You will remain unlucky if that is your belief system. The true lesson comes from awareness, then applying energy or action to the situation to move away from it. That energy is a spark of the inspiration energy field. It is always there to access.

Shamans have direct access to these energy fields. They can alter their physical bodies in a way to surpass the density and enter into the fields of love, inspiration and divine perfection. There are also lower energetic fields. None of which are bad or evil, just lower vibrations. These consist of fear, and envy and grief. Humans experience all of these within a human lifetime, except the ascended masters who remained in higher vibrational states. All humans or souls can experience pieces of each vibration. It is based on sheer will and awareness that you can navigate through each field and pull your vibration higher so you can move to a more pleasant state of being.

Shamans hold ancient wisdom. The ancients knew this information. They knew how to move through energy fields while still living a human experience. Many of the rituals or ceremonies held by the shaman are to make the soul remember how to overcome its boundaries. Once the soul can surpass the boundary of dense matter, body, it is open to all fields of energy. Shamanic tradition /wisdom, holds this knowledge. It can help humans live a more fulfilled human experience. It can help souls feel more connected and whole. Shamanism opens humans' eyes to the interconnectedness of all beings. All creations, energy and matter. Even still, or non "alive" matter holds vibrations. This is evident in minerals and crystals.

The shaman removes the veil of ignorance and separation. Shamanic practices are important but not necessary. It is just a means to finding wholeness and communicating with the larger body or energetic field.

Talk to me about the human link to true inspiration and God creation.

Inspiration is a way of the soul birthing something into physical form. Inspiration is a vibration. You can tap into this vibration and feel inspiration course through your entire body. Once attuned to inspiration it flows through the physical body creating motivation and sparking idea into form. We see this all the time. Everything that ever was that is human made was once a thought. That human tapped into the divine frequency of inspiration and received the energy or motivation to move forward and birth their project into form. This is very similar as to how all souls are created.

The divine source was inspired to birth each and every piece of itself into form. It is not true that source was lonely. There is no such thing as loneliness in Divine Perfection. Source had no other choice as to expand, being its natural state. With this expansion came the frequency of inspiration. With inspiration came the desire to manifest into form. This is a cycle that each and every human participates in on earth. Inspiration to create, to nurture, to teach, it all comes from connecting with this frequency.

TWENTY-FIVE MESSAGES
FOR HUMANITY

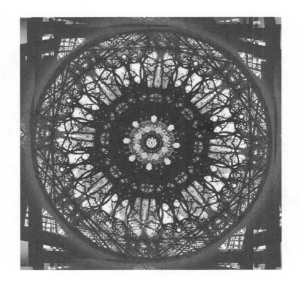

"I decided that it was not wisdom that enabled poets to write their poetry, but a kind of instinct or inspiration, such as you find in seers and prophets who deliver all their sublime messages without knowing in the least what they mean."
- Socrates

Message 1

The sounds of others voices are vibrations of their soul. It is important that everyone learn the song of their soul. Each song is unique and perfect, just like a snowflake. That is why you are so sensitive to sound. The vibrations echo a familiar song in your heart. You can connect to each vibration by manipulating yours to match it. Even though you can match your vibration with others, it doesn't mean you should always do it. Let the vibrations either flow through you or bounce off of you, don't absorb them. Feel the vibrations and radiate them. Let them guide you always.

Message 2

You are a book that is constantly being rewritten. Do not hold yourself to any standards or rules, let go of expectations and be present.

Message 3

You are a beautiful masterpiece of DNA, love, time and stardust. Celebrate your magic!

Message 4

You can accomplish anything you dream. Do not let doubt or fears block you from being a master of your own life and its creations.

Message 5

Have faith in all that is good. Everything will work out exactly as it is supposed to.

Message 6

Trust your gut always, you are the keeper and mastermind to all of your decisions.

Message 7

Keep your space sacred. You are the master of all objects and beings who can enter it.

Message 8

You are the giver of beauty and joy to many who surround you.

Message 9

Keep your thoughts positive about yourself and others. You are powerful and so are your words.

Message 10

Dance. Dance now & often, have fun move and laugh.

Message 11

Prepare for the Best, Expect the Best and you WILL Manifest the Best.

Message 12

Create.

Message 13

Have fun, always every day and in everything.

Message 14

Don't take everything so seriously.

Message 15

Let go of expectations.

Message 16

When life gets rough, ride the wave, see where it brings you.

Message 17

Always explore, your emotions and internal world as well as your external physical world.

Message 18

Free up your time, space and obligations.

Message 19

Find time for stillness every day.

Message 20

Change the System within yourself.

You can change the system within yourself by not working too hard to be taken seriously or rewarded. Be still. In stillness you will find the answers and the strength. Stop, say no, be still be still be still. Rest your body let go of the push to succeed. You are already there. You have succeeded. You found your truth in the darkest storm. You have activated the light and now allow it to lead you. Do not worry or fear. Trust, flow stillness. Do not overthink your future. Easily and effortlessly move into it. Surrender. You have been unbound. Unwound and unrestrained.

Message 21

You are a supreme being of light and form. You are meant to experience both. Do not get caught up in either world. Live in your body to the fullest experiencing emotions and physical sensations. Create joy when you are hopeless, peace when you are anxious and love when you are fearful. You are a master creator. Channel your light and transmute low vibrations into higher ones. You have that ability and power. You will feel the results in your cells. Have faith that you can transmute anything into goodness.

Message 22

Wait until you feel completely set in your ways and then shake them up. Never become attached to any particular way of being.

Release rules and allow yourself to be open. Move away from expectations and attachments.

Message 23

You do not owe anyone anything in this life except yourself. Be true to you and all the best for you. Never let another's voice overpower yours. Speak and you will be free.

Message 24

Stay in the now as much as possible. If the mind wanders, bring it back with the senses. Enjoy the sensations that you have been gifted in this body.

Message 25

Perpetuate Peace.

GODDESS SPEAK

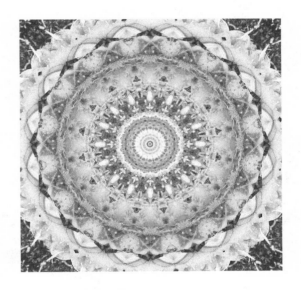

"I have called on the Goddess and found her within myself"
— Marion Zimmer Bradley, The Mists of Avalon

I *am opening myself up to new dimensions now. Dimensions of my sacred soul. The high priestess medicine woman that I am and came here to be. I follow with love and trust and work towards a goal of peace.*

Women and men everywhere, sacred sisters and brothers, follow your callings now as I have, to speak the truth of our souls and our cells. No longer will we be burned for the truth. Stifled not. Go! Go out into the world and do your work but first you must find your peace and solidarity to Thyself.

Today is the first day of the rest of your life.

Daily mantra: <u>*Piece together the confusion to find clarity.*</u> <u>*Calm the longing with wisdom. Stop the lonely suffering with*</u> <u>*community. Peace, Peace, Peace.*</u>

Rise up now and fill your heart with all that it desires. Let go of the pain from the sisters and brothers of the past. Heal the wound of persecution and rise up. Today is the day. Every little step is important. There is not an end goal, only a constant evolution of spirit.

Durga I call unto thee. What lessons do you have for me? Durga, high priestess of my tribe. I bow unto your feet and ask for your help in showing me the way.

Durga: Beautiful Goddess of the East

Many hands are not for producing but for giving. Service can only be successful if you have something to give. You can only have something to give if your cup is full. Do not let the power of having many roles fool you. You cannot be everything and anything all at once. Surrender into your flow and allow each hand to support and hold you. Surrender into being held. Held by me, others and yourself. Hold yourself dearly and feel that support you can give yourself. It's time to let go now of all ideals and things that are just not a match for your energy. You will see those things that lower your vibrations. Why are you sick? What energetic pieces did you sacrifice? Rest, rest, rest. I will always be here.

I had just been reborn. Unexpected events have led to a rather beautiful climax. I gave up, surrendered to the universe and allowed myself to be reborn. I was instructed to do a baptism of sorts. I cried tears and wailed out loud as I drew the bath. I surrender I surrender I surrender. I was intuitively instructed to collect ingredients. Orange peels, sea salt, lavender, tea tree, frankincense and black spruce oils & holy water from the river Jordan. I was also called to grab my largest crystals and submerged myself into the bath. Spirit speaks.

Spirit wants me to know:

You did it beauty, you let go of control. Walk for ever more with the grace and confidence your eternal soul possesses. Fear not doubt not. You are never alone. We are here as the ban of sisters and brothers to guide you through this life. You can now clearly hear our voices sing unto thee. No more drowning out our cries. Hooray and welcome to the first day of the rest of your life. You have no idea how much beauty you bring into the world. You are a powerful manifestor. Hold onto this. You can birth ANYTHING into being just by pondering it up. Now it is time to do the real work. So much beauty awaits. Freedom at last! You are one of the leaders in this movement. No time to waste or to dim your light. Feel this coolness around you, that is the power of She. Follow her flow. Flow with her always and all of your needs will be met. So excited for you my love. Keep going up and up and up and up. The next step will be presented soon. Eyes wide open you will know what to do. So much love surrounds you now and always. Keep that love frequency as a navigation tool. Love peace and joy all with flow and ease. Any discomfort is your sign to move away. You have birthed you have felt the twinges of labor and all of the pain. Now it's time to really be born. Be alive fully alive. Remember eyes wide open and ears. Hear our whispers. We no longer need to shout. You are in tune and in perfect alignment to hear us. Love you beautiful child and powerful goddess. Keep changing the world.

Thank you, Dear Ones who guide me, always <3

COMING HOME

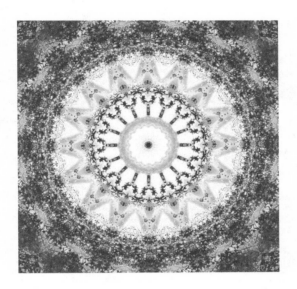

"Every day is a journey, and the journey itself is home."
- Matsuo Basho

Go around the world and navigate your life with peace in your heart, mind, body and soul. Do not get frustrated over the insignificant details. Allow peace to be the vibration you echo to all souls you encounter and that peace will be returned to you.

Love one another no matter how hard it gets at times. Love is the essence of all, no matter what your mind tells you. Love first, next and always. Love really is the key to any anguish you feel. How can you love yourself and all those around you to your best ability? Love means no judgement, or expectations. Love means service and devotion to you highest calling. Love means peace and peace means love.

The whispers of the unsung tails float within reachable distance. You are all susceptible to the lore of the ancients and ascended beings. Reach above your illusionary visions to process the expansive nature of your true essence.

It isn't the daily grind or desire that makes you human, it is the aspiration to achieve. Humans must expand. The methods chosen can either be destructive or beneficial to the whole. Look upon your footprints and read within them the tale of your own expansive nature.

Methods such as yoga have been passed onto you so you can move beyond the illusionary form of matter and find union with your ultimate vibration.

Fear not about the path that unfolds. Walk with eyes open and take in the sights along the way with the senses. Do not succumb to the drama created by your mind. Allow peace to fill your being at every moment.

Use the tools supplied many moons ago to connect you back to home.

Move through your incarnation with grace and ease. The human struggle is an illusion. Comfort is always available by moving within.

Treat others with respect as they move through their own confusing journey. Only they can unravel the veil that they pulled before their own eyes. Do not disrupt their process. The ones who want to learn will come to the. All others will perpetuate the patterns they have fallen into.

Do not get trapped by the material. It is unnecessary and will be distracting on your quest to enlightenment.

Surrender into the flow of the universe. Allow the spinning of the planets and cycles of the moon to pull you.

Be free my child, be free, be free be free.